# Multiple Sclerosis? You can do it!

Ewout van den Engel

# Multiple Sclerosis? You can do it!

Overcoming multiple sclerosis in practice

2020 MKBsocial

**Multiple Sclerosis? You can do it!**
**Overcoming multiple sclerosis in practice**
ISBN: 9798682777075
All rights reserved (2019/2020)
Author: Ewout van den Engel
Publisher: MKBsocial, Heerlen
Want to use content from this book? Contact us at
www.mkbsocial.nl
Translated from Dutch, original title:
Multiple sclerose? Zet 'm op! Multiple sclerose
overwinnen doe je zo.

## With special thanks to

Rose for the help with the translation to English.

The following fantastic people for helping me with the translation of the dinner cards in the annex: Aysu, Belghin, Bogi, Gabriel, Gabriel D., Calliopi, Michele, Mihail, Miho, Morteza, Nkolay, Olga, Rawan, Romy, Sarka, Sigrid.

# Table of contents

## *Foreword*

Every year, tens of thousands of people are diagnosed with MS worldwide. The diagnosis is primarily a curse: you lose not only control over your life, but also control over your body. However, the disease can also be a blessing, at least it was for me. Adopting the Overcoming Multiple Sclerosis (OMS) lifestyle gave me hope and as we say in Dutch; hoop doet leven; hope makes life. In this booklet I want to share with you the experience I have had with (O) MS for the last 10 years. It's important to note that what I have written refers to my own experience. Where necessary, I have indicated supporting sources. You are probably already familiar with the principles of Overcoming Multiple Sclerosis and you may have already read the book Overcoming Multiple Sclerosis. Still, just to be sure, I highlight the OMS program in the chapter About (O) MS.

Just as the shoemaker sticks to their trade, I don't make statements that go beyond my experience. I have never used medicine to treat multiple sclerosis myself and I am not a doctor or a pharmacist, so I can't tell you anything useful about this. The same applies to preparations such as cannabis oil, eating habits such as intermittent fasting and other alternative therapies. All I can tell you about this is that there is no magic pill or miracle method. Overcoming MS takes a lot of effort and a long time before you see results, but they are real and lasting. All you need is time, discipline and a bit of stubbornness. I hope that the advice in this book will help you and that you come back to this e-book to refresh your memory. MS? You can do it!

Ewout van den Engel

*Remember that all advice has been given from my personal experience and is not mandatory. Everything in this release is for informational purposes only. Nothing is intended as medical advice and should not be interpreted as such.*

## A little more about (O) MS

The OMS program is based on the book Overcoming Multiple Sclerosis: An Evidence-based Guide to Recovery by the Australian professor and physician George Jelinek, first published in 2000. OMS is a series of guidelines based on the study of more than 70,000 scientific articles on MS. Scientific research has long pointed to a link between your lifestyle and its consequences on your health. A western lifestyle, i.e. lack of exercise, and (too much) fat, dairy, meat, frying, etc., is strongly associated with most diseases of affluence, like most cancers, diabetes and MS. If you follow the OMS program strictly (and that is the only way), you will start feeling better after about three months, with attacks generally subsiding after nine to twelve months. Sometimes it can take up to three years before attacks start subsiding, but after five years you will be generally stable.

## Summary of (O) MS

### Diet and Supplements

- A plant-based diet with fish, avoiding saturated and processed fats.
- Daily intake of 20 grams of omega-3 oil in the form

of flaxseed or fish oil, or up to 40 grams if you lead an active lifestyle (a tablespoon is about 10 grams).

- If necessary, B group vitamins or vitamin B12 supplements.

## Vitamin D

- Vitamin D3 supplement of 5000 IU -10,000 IU per day. Focus on a blood value of 150nmol / L or 60ng/mL and above. On days with moderate to very strong UV index, you can also suffice with sunbathing until your skin becomes slightly coloured; note that your body must be predominantly uncovered.

## Meditation

- 30 minutes a day.

## Sports / intensive exercise

- 30 continuous minutes each day, preferably 5 times a week.

## Medicines

- In consultation with your neurologist if waiting is not an option. OMS does not exclude medication; it is based on the premise of 'do whatever it takes'.

## The role of milk protein

Nobody knows exactly how MS arises, but it is agreed that your body's immune system attacks its own nervous system. This attack is associated with the presence of certain milk proteins[1]. In MS, the nerve pathways in your

---

[1] See overcomingms.org/recovery-program/diet/dairy-and-ms

spine and brain are attacked, but your nervous system runs throughout your whole body, sending amongst others messages to your muscles so you can hold your pee. Simply put, a signal runs from your brain through your spinal cord to your bladder muscle.

Now, imagine your nervous system as an electrical cable surrounded by a plastic insulation layer. In your body, that insulation is formed by the fatty substance called myelin. When that myelin is attacked and becomes damaged, the signals from your brain can no longer reach your bladder muscle without being disturbed. This leads to you nor being able to hold you pee.

One of the reasonings behind the OMS program is that if you stop eating or drinking products containing milk protein, eventually, there will be no 'foreign' milk protein in your body. This means that the immune system is no longer stimulated to attack the myelin, allowing for a rest in which the myelin can slowly recover.

## The role of fats

It is best for your immune system if in your body there's a balance between omega-6 and omega-3 fats. Most people have an imbalance between the two because of their eating habits: they consume too much omega-6 (for example from sunflower oil and seeds) and too little omega-3 (for example from fish)[2]. While omega-3 calms your immune system, omega-6 does the exact opposite. An imbalance between omega 6 and omega 3 is e.g. 15:1,

---

[2] See ncbi.nlm.nih.gov/pubmed/12442909

while a healthy ratio is around 5:1 or lower. Eating (products containing) omega-3 fat daily and avoiding products containing processed omega-6 fat will slowly restore the omega-3 / omega-6 balance in your body so your immune system will be less likely to overreact to an intruder.

In addition, there is another important advantage. Your body, as you know, is made up of cells. These cells all have a cell membrane which consists mostly of fat. If there is inflammation in your body, the inflamed cells will swell, much like we see with a swollen finger. Because the inflamed cells swell, they will press on the surrounding healthy cells. MS involves inflammation of cells in your brain and spinal cord. A cell membrane consisting of saturated fat is not flexible and bursts under pressure. However, a cell membrane that is made up of omega-3 will instead bend and therefore will not burst. As a result, inflammation does less (surrounding) damage if the cell membranes are made up of omega-3 fat rather than saturated (omega-6) fat.

## Download leaflets

Do you want to know more about the OMS program, for example about the effects of meditation or movement? Then download the leaflets at overcomingms.org/resources/free-downloads.

## *Keep a diary*

It usually takes a long time before it is clear that you have
MS. I think in my case it may have taken a year and a
half with symptoms on and off. First was the signal from
Lhermitte[3] in the spring of 2009. At the end of the
summer, I had a period in which I had vision and balance
issues. In the winter I felt numb from my lower leg to my
lower back. Finally, at the end of the following summer I
was experiencing spasms, a speech impediment, tingling
in my torso, the soles of my feet, hand and arm and
more. An MRI followed and the diagnosis was made. With
all these symptoms separately I always thought: ah, it's
just a one-time inconvenience or I must have slept badly.
The reason I remember all this is that I started to keep a
blog after diagnosis. A diary is of course also a good
alternative.

To properly prepare the upcoming conversations
with your neurologist and to check the course of your
symptoms, it is useful to keep a diary. Start by writing
down any symptoms you can remember. You can do this
together with someone close to you who may remember
when you had a complaint about something or when you

---

[3] This is an electrical current felt in the spinal cord.

felt tired. State exactly what you experienced and when, for example 'June 2017 around the 18th: pressing pain in my arm lasting about 2 weeks.' If you are unsure whether something has to do with MS, please mention it anyway. After you describe the past, you begin the present. Describe everything you find worth mentioning, even if you think your symptoms or state of mind may be due to something else. You will gradually begin to describe the course of your illness.

Now the underlying idea comes: once every few months (six months is best) you can read the development of your disease and you can reflect on the course of your MS. You don't have to be afraid of this. If you commit to the OMS lifestyle, your quality of life will improve anyway, even if it's only the small inconveniences that stay away. What you will probably see is that complaints disappear, the attacks decrease and you feel better. An easy way to analyze your diary is to assign a number or a color to every month. This way you can quickly see how your quality of life has changed over time. Don't forget to mention the good things too!

### Keep in mind

✓ First describe the past, then the present.
✓ Also mention positive experiences: good food, first time exercise and the progress of this.
✓ If you are unsure whether something has to do with MS, write it down!
✓ Read your diary before going to the neurologist. This way you can discuss doubts, but also provide them with accurate information.

## *Reading food labels*

The first time going shopping on the OMS lifestyle was a disaster for me. I had to reinvent my shopping habits and read labels madly. It turned out that it only made sense to visit certain aisles in the supermarket and ignore other ones by default. During that period I entered an ecological supermarket or a health food store for the first time, which have now become trusted places. Surprisingly, I find many products there that also do not fit into the OMS lifestyle because they contain organic palm oil or coconut oil. I noticed that you only really know whether a product is healthy for you, if you learn to read the label on the back of the packet.

On the back of the packet there are two types of information: the nutritional values and the ingredients. You need to study them both and also check them regularly for changes. Manufacturers sometimes want to change the ingredients of a product over time. There is no particular order to read a packet.

### Nutrition facts

With the nutrition label, you are interested in the 'total fat, saturated' per serving size. In my experience, the number here must be less than a gram, otherwise I won't even read on. You can immediately put all products with a content of above one gram back on the shelf, with the exception of products based on olives, avocado, fish or with extra-virgin oil added. In the case of cocoa (powder / beans) I do take into account the amount of saturated fat. You don't have to pay attention to the part 'carbohydrates, total sugars', but eating too much added sugar does not fit into a healthy lifestyle. 50 to 60 grams of sugar is the maximum daily intake recommended by the World Health Organization.

## Ingredients

When looking at the ingredients label, the first rule to remember is that the ingredients are ordered by quantity: the first ingredient has the highest amount. This is useful to know if it concerns ingredients that you should not strictly avoid, but which are not healthy in large quantities. Think of glucose fructose syrup[4] and refined sugars or in the case of exceptional situations (see Finding options when there are none). If the label only lists ingredients that fit the OMS lifestyle, but the saturated fat is higher than I gram, you can still eat it because the saturated fat then comes from products such as olives, avocado and oily fish.

Note, sometimes certain oils are not listed on the label. If a product feels greasy, it probably contains fat. For example, I once bought falafel for the (microwave) oven which didn't contain fat according to the ingredients, but felt greasy. After eating this falafel a few times, I started to have doubts and sent an e-mail to the

---

[4] Also known as glucose syrup and fructose syrup.

manufacturer. They told me casually that the falafel briefly passed through a bath of hot oil after preparation. So if it feels greasy, it probably contains fat and it's better to skip the product next time.

## A few more general remarks

- If possible, avoid mono- and diglycerides of fatty acids (usually used as an emulsifier in bread, under ingredients).
- Oil: cold pressed oil[5] or (extra) virgin. If one of these statements is not listed, avoid the product.
- Organic oil: avoid organic oil if it does not mention that it is cold pressed.

## Keep in mind

- ✓ Never trust the front of the package, always read the label on the back.
- ✓ On the nutrition label, saturated fat and sugars are good indications of whether a product is healthy or not.
- ✓ Ingredients are listed in order of quantity.
- ✓ Sometimes there can be hidden fat in a product.
- ✓ Irrespective of what is written on the label, if a product feels greasy or tastes fatty, it probably contains (unmentioned) fat.

---

[5] All cold-pressed oils, except for coconut oil and palm oil, fall within OMS, but you must take care that you do not consume too many omega-6 fats (for example, cold-pressed sunflower oil). If you have the choice, opt for cold-pressed olive oil.

# *Excercise*

Accepting your MS as part of your life and as part of yourself is tough. But accepting a dire situation, resolves the stress from not coming to terms with it. Want to try a little exposure therapy? Get a pencil or pen and fill up this page with as many repetitions of "I accept my MS' as possible.

# Finding options when there are none

A question you often hear is: can I have cheat days? The answer is absolutely not. Cheating means cutting corners, deliberately ignoring guidelines or coming up with your own exceptions. But is there really no deviation possible? This question brings me to a sensitive point, because I have experienced situations in which I was very hungry, without a real OMS choice or where I had strong doubts about what I was presented with. It was and remains to be a personal choice of what you allow for yourself in such circumstances. I have always weighed my choices against the principles of Overcoming Multiple Sclerosis and the practical side that Roy Swank explained in his book Multiple Sclerosis Diet Book, one of the foundations of OMS. Remember: this is what I do in exceptional situations. This chapter gives you advice, which by definition differs from OMS.

Let's first look at the main principles of OMS about food:

1) The less saturated fat from animal products an MS patient eats, the more favorable the course of their MS.

2) It is very likely that your immune system reacts offensively to milk protein, which is absorbed into

the insulation layer of your nervous system.
3) An imbalance of omega-3 and omega-6 levels causes an overactive immune system.
4) Processed oil, such as refined sunflower oil, causes bad cell membranes.
5) Do not eat meat.

What does this mean for emergencies?

There is almost no saturated fat in skinned poultry (e.g. chicken or turkey breast) and in principle, it fits within OMS, although the book strictly states no meat. Meat is not part of OMS for two reasons:
1) Excessive meat consumption has been linked to various diseases, such as cancer.
2) OMS is clearer this way. Otherwise you get a bunch of exceptions, endless discussions (why not kangaroo meat? Etc.) and a slippery slope of justifications (but if chicken breast is possible, why not some lean pork? And if lean pork is possible, why not a steak? Etc.).

In case of an emergency, you can therefore eat (grilled) chicken or turkey breast without any problems.

A second thing that you run into when there are no OMS options is the use of (sunflower) oil, which is often incorporated into foods. Choose the option with the least amount of oil possible and remove as much of it as you can with a napkin. Never opt for fried food. As a guideline and for reassurance: half a tablespoon of refined sunflower oil per year is nothing compared to the 730 tablespoons of omega-3 oil that you take per year following the OMS diet. However, don't let it be more than half a tablespoon or a teaspoon. Always try to avoid milk protein.

## Keep in mind

✓ The OMS diet is all about avoiding milk protein and saturated fat from animal products.
✓ Eating (grilled or boiled) lean, white meat such as chicken or turkey breast won't hurt as a one off.
✓ Always try to remove as much oil as possible.
✓ 'Prefer' vegetable oil over milk protein.

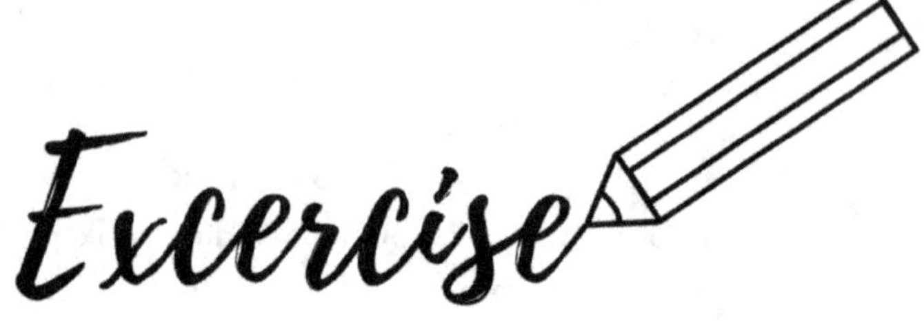

When we are hungry we get stressed and when we get stressed we think less clear and are more prone to bad nutritional decisions. To prevent this from happening keep hydrated. Also make sure you always have some snacks available to you at home and on the go. Think of six OMS friendly snacks that are available to you in your local supermarket or easy to get by on the go:

1)

2)

3)

4)

5)

6)

(Examples: bananas, avocado, raw nuts, carrots, smoked fish etc.)

## Sports: focus on the long run

Before I got MS, I ran 8-15 kilometers at a time, two to three times a week. After my worst attack, which eventually led to a visit to the neurologist and the diagnosis, I couldn't even run to the end of the street. Soon after the symptoms of the attack subsided, I started running again but it was trial and error. On the days when I was feeling fit, I would go for a jog with the aim of completing 3 - 4 km., but I often had to give up somewhere around halfway. Only about 20 months after starting the OMS lifestyle was I able to jog six to eight kilometers once or twice a week. I also went swimming for an hour a couple of times a week. Now, more than ten years after the diagnosis, I exercise about twice a week and occasionally hike in the Romanian mountains.

Whether you have been exercising before your diagnosis or want to start after your diagnosis, in both cases you will often have to start at zero. MS has damaged your nervous system and thus damaged the nerve paths previously used for signals for movement. With repeated attempts to move, you stimulate your body to create a diversion in your nervous system. This ensures that the movement can still be carried out in the long term. The trick with sports is to never go beyond your limits and always listen carefully to your body. While exercising, constantly ask yourself the questions: Is it getting too much? Do I feel I'm going too far? Can I barely keep it up? If you answer yes to one of the questions, stop at that point or at least ease off a bit. The goal is not to finish one training, but to be able to start the next.

Rather than setting goals based on distance or number of training sessions, instead focus on the time you invest. Remember: all movement counts! So also shuffleboard, chess or jeu de boules. Anything to train your nervous system to move in a coordinated way is good. It's preferable to exercise for 30 minutes continuously, three to five times a week. This can also be done in two fifteen minute blocks a day. It is not a disaster if you cannot achieve what you set out to do, or what you could do before MS. Do what you can and you will see that you will progress in small steps. In that respect it is nice to include this routine in your diary. This way you can see your progress over the months. You can view all activities that require intensive exercise as a sport[6], such as cycling to work or the supermarket.

In terms of nutrition, you don't have to do anything extraordinary before exercising. Make sure you have eaten in advance but do not exercise on a full stomach (wait an hour before starting). Depending on the intensity, it is important to start drinking water (up to 1 liter) about an hour and a half in advance. Don't wait

---

[6] I have specifically checked this with OMS. Also see overcomingms.org/recovery-program/exercise/what-are-my-exercise-options

until you're already doing sports. On days when you do intensive exercise, it is important to take a bit more omega-3 oil than usual, approximately one tablespoon more.

Eating a banana right after exercise can counteract muscle pain due to the carbohydrate content. Also, make sure you don't overheat. In addition to drinking water in advance, I recommend adjusting your pace in the case of outdoor sports at high temperatures. For example, you can start exercising early in the morning, between 6am and 9am to avoid exercising during hotter times of the day. If you are unable to do your regular exercises for a day, try another form of exercise that works or take a day off. The aim is to move for a better quality of life; not (yet) to climb Mount Everest.

### Keep in mind

- ✓ After your diagnosis you will have to start from scratch.
- ✓ Ease off during exercise if you feel it is becoming too much.
- ✓ Exercise based on time, not distance or number of training sessions.
- ✓ Record your exercise routine in your diary.
- ✓ Do not exercise on an empty or full stomach and eat a banana afterwards.
- ✓ Take some more omega-3 oil on the days when you exercise.
- ✓ If it's not working on a given day, try something else or take a rest day.

# Excercise

Stimulating your cognition (training your brain), can be done as silly or as serious as you want it to be. You can start doing puzzles, learn a new language or just learn how to do the 'Vulcan Salute' with both hands. Or have you tried moving your small toes outward lately?

## Learning to meditate

I can still remember the first meditations after the diagnosis. I would come home from work, change into comfortable clothes and lie on my bed for half an hour. Then, for thirty minutes, all kinds of thoughts raced through my head, while I was trying hard to focus on an imaginary dot in the middle of my forehead. In the first weeks it was still not going well, but I soon found a technique that worked for me: inhale deeply through your nose and exhale carefully through your mouth. This allowed me to experience for the first time a short silence between breaths. Later that silence grew a little longer and I noticed how I could hear the birds chirping outside. From that time on, I also used meditation to calm myself periodically. In itself, however, this is not so useful if you do not also tackle the source of the stress.

I personally benefited from the book The Power of Now[7] by Eckhart Tolle, of which I would read a number of pages every day. I then reflected on what I read and tried to apply the advice immediately. Eckhart Tolle actually propagates a form of mindfulness, which

---

[7] The Power Of Now has a spiritual side. You don't necessarily have to pay attention to that part.

more or less corresponds to meditating throughout the day. You start living on the principle that you live in the present: the only time frame that you can influence. The past has already happened, so you can't change that anymore. The future is yet to come, so you can't do anything with that either. From these observations, several wisdoms follow:

**Past**: If you experience (emotional) problems from the past, try to solve them. Forgive people unilaterally, accept that you cannot change the past and also dare to accept that you can never be fully blamed for anything. There are always multiple parties involved in a conflict, sometimes bearing more responsibility than you. Also accept that you are no longer the same person as you were then.

You cannot take responsibility for anything that happened in your childhood, because you were a child and a child cannot see all the consequences. Parents can do that much better, for example, but they are also merely people of flesh and blood who do not hold the truth.

**Future**: It is of no use to think about all kinds of unlikely future scenarios. The future will not turn out that way. Your concerns about the future are actually projections of your concerns in the present.

**Present**: In the now you can change something, work on your emotional state and learn to accept things. If you are in an (emotionally) unpleasant situation, you have three options to do something about it: accept the situation, try to change the situation or leave the situation.

To ensure that you no longer think about the

past and the future (and thus pay more attention to the present), Eckhart Tolle suggests that you intensively observe your own thoughts. You need to become aware of your thoughts and realize that you are not your thoughts. You also exist without thoughts and still have a character.

You consciously deal with your thoughts by categorizing every thought that 'comes in' as about the past or about the future. Then you say to yourself: 'not relevant'. At first, it will take you a while to realize that you are lost in thought, but with enough work, you will move forward. So far forward that you will be able to cut them off at the beginning or sometimes won't even have them at all. What remains is space and silence in your head. If you come across thoughts that keep coming back, write them down but don't stop there. Keep writing to find where that thought came from. Recurring thoughts indicate unresolved problems or fears that you are not facing. On a side note: You will have to get used to the newfound silence in your head, but you can use that space to focus more on the outside world or to pay more attention to others.

### Keep in mind

- ✓ There are different methods of meditation. The main thing is to get peace of mind.
- ✓ You are not your thoughts.
- ✓ Try to cut off thoughts about the past and the future as quickly as possible.
- ✓ Also don't forget to tackle the source of your anxiety.
- ✓ Read The Power of Now carefully and apply what you read right away. Read page by page, spread over several weeks.

# Excercise

Close your eyes for a moment. Breathe in deep through your mouth. Keep the air in your lungs for a second and release it through your mouth again. Repeat and try to keep in the air for two seconds now and release. Continue and try to find your own rhythm. As you start to relax focus your hearing on one particular sound around you. Keep the focus until your eyes open by themselves.

## *Choosing a suitable restaurant*

One of the best books I have ever read about living with an MS diet is R.L. Swank's book: Multiple Sclerosis Diet Book. Although outdated, it is very useful. It not only addresses the background of MS, but also Swank's own study of 150 MS patients on a fat-free diet over a span of more than 30 years[8]. The most helpful part was about eating out. I will be elaborating on Swank's tips in this chapter. Honor where credit is due.

I prepared the following dinner card (next page) which usually offers enough guidance in a restaurant, but can also be used when you eat with friends. You will find translations of the card in more than twenty foreign languages in the annex, so you can travel with confidence.

## Advice for restaurant visits

Always try to book in advance and explain your diet. Use the dinner card for this and always ask for a menu proposal. It is best to choose restaurants in the middle and upper price range as these restaurants can better accommodate your dietary needs. Cheaper restaurants that usually work with standard menus often cannot

---

[8] See swankmsdiet.org/about-the-swank-ms-foundation

accommodate you well. If you are invited to a dinner with work or friends, make sure the person making the reservation has the necessary information by forwarding them the dinner card.

Hello!

I follow a strict medical diet. Are you able to cook me something?

I can't eat products with:

- Processed / refined oils
- Meat
- Dairy (milk, butter, etc)
- Egg yolk
- (Deep) fried foods
- Coconut

I can have, among others:

- ✓ Fish
- ✓ Vegetables, fruit, nuts
- ✓ Pasta, bread, rice
- ✓ Extra virgin olive oil
- ✓ Other cold-pressed oils

Possible modes of preparation:

- ✓ Grilled, in the oven, steamed, boiled

Thank you!

*Dinner card*

If you do not make a reservation, let the waiter know immediately that you are following a strict medical diet by means of the dinner card. Do not be rushed by other customers and don't be afraid to bother your waiter, they're there to help you. Sometimes my first sentence is even: 'I may be your most annoying customer of the evening.'

Keep in mind that you will consume hidden oils at any restaurant, especially since you never have 100% control over the preparation and what mood the chef is in that day. As a rule, do not eat out more than once a week. It is also preferable not to use a salad dressing if it is unclear what oil it contains.

If you have a choice between the type of restaurant or kitchen, I recommend to choose or avoid the following places:

**Choose**: Seafood restaurants / Japanese (sushi) / Italian / Spanish / French / vegetarian / vegan * / Mediterranean / Moroccan.
**Avoid**: Fast food restaurants / snack bars / the local fish & chips shop / kebab stall / hamburger restaurants / grill restaurants / Mexican / Chinese / Indonesian / typically Belgian / typically German.

* Note: coconut and sunflower oil is frequently used in vegan and raw vegan restaurants. There is also a lot of fried food in vegan restaurants, so don't order on the assumption that it will be in line with the OMS diet.

### Keep in mind

✓ Print the dinner card and put it in your wallet, so you always have it ready. Also make sure you have a digital version on your phone so that you can always forward it to friends or a restaurant.

✓ If you do not make the reservation yourself, please inform the organization in advance of your dietary requirements.

✓ Choose restaurants in the middle or upper price range.

✓ Watch out for coconut oil and refined sunflower oil at so-called (raw) vegan restaurants.

✓ Try not to eat out more than once a week.

## *Prepare for travel*

Every time I travel, I worry about the hotel breakfast, lunch and dinner. I have noticed that preparation is essential. Even so, you still need a back-up plan. For example, I once called ahead to a hotel to ask if they had soy milk for breakfast. They confirmed that they did and sure enough, when I actually was at the breakfast buffet during my trip, the milk wasn't there. The next day it was, but the third day again it wasn't. That didn't matter that much anymore, because I had bought just soy milk myself already. I also base this chapter partly on the tips of R.L. Swank from Multiple Sclerosis Diet Book.

When traveling, breakfast will be one of your major concerns; you wake up and you feel hungry. When you stay at a guest house, bed & breakfast or local hotel, breakfast is often limited, traditional and not OMS friendly. Therefore, always try to bring your own breakfast for the first day. Think of soy milk, oatmeal, dried fruit, hummus and bread or a homemade, savory biscuit. I myself often bring a plastic bowl and a spoon to make my own breakfast, if I think there won't be any at the property.

If you stay in a hotel with several stars, you will often have an 'intercontinental' breakfast buffet. You will always find a boiled egg, which you can eat without the yolk with bread. There may also be extra-virgin olive oil that you can sprinkle over it. Some breakfast buffets also offer smoked fish and salad, and there is always jam, toast, fruit and corn flakes. Always ask for soy milk or other plant-based milk. Note that some vegetable milk also contains oil, so ask for the packaging if possible to double check. In this case, your back-up breakfast will help.

If your hotel has a fridge in the room, you can store flaxseed oil and other food that you take with you. You can always ask for a fridge if there isn't one in the room, or maybe you can keep something in the fridge of the accommodation itself. If you are traveling for a long time, check in advance whether you can buy linseed oil anywhere on location. You can also choose to bring fish oil capsules or cans of oily fish. With linseed oil capsules you will have to check with the manufacturer whether the oil is cold pressed.

To find good places to eat and health food stores, you can use the Happy Cow app in most countries. In addition, you can always search on Google Maps for, for example, an Italian restaurant nearby or one of the other suitable cuisines. In the annex you will find translations of the earlier mentioned dinner card. You can also use this card in the supermarket if you are not sure about the ingredients in a product. You then only have to point to the label and then to the paragraph I can't eat products with in the language in question.

### Keep in mind
✓ Always call ahead and inquire about breakfast.

- ✓ Bring an emergency breakfast.
- ✓ Ask for a fridge.
- ✓ Download the Happy Cow app and use Google Maps.
- ✓ Consult the annex with the translations of the dinner cards.
- ✓ See also the chapters Finding options when there are none and Choosing a suitable restaurant.

# Excercise

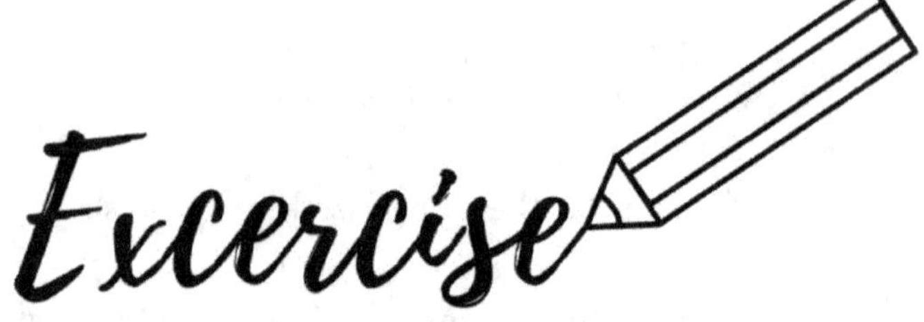

Many restaurants have dishes that can be slightly altered to cater to your needs. Think about:

- ☺ Tuna salad (leave out the egg)
- ☺ Pasta arrabiata (no cheese, no or very little refined oil)
- ☺ Pizza (leave out the cheese and ask for extra tomato sauce)
- ☺ Boiled or steamed vegetables (no butter)
- ☺ Fish (no oil or butter)

Think about your favorite restaurant. What dishes that only need slight altering could you still enjoy?

## Build a good relationship with your neurologist

My relationship with my neurologist was very problematic. It was probably not so much his fault, but more my fighting spirit and suspicion about his advice which was unjustified, because after all he was only doing his job. I always wanted to convince my neurologist that I was right, that a diet low in saturated fat works for people with multiple sclerosis. In fact I did this because at the time I was still unsure whether it would all work. The turbulent history with my neurologist is echoed in the firmness with which I wrote this chapter.

For a good relationship with your neurologist it is important to know what you can expect from them (and what not to expect). A neurologist is a physician who specializes in diseases of the nervous system, such as Parkinson's, Alzheimer's and MS. The neurologist knows how the nervous system works and is aware of the usual treatments. In the case of MS, we talk about treatment with medication. Neurologists, like all physicians, are liable for their work and therefore prefer not to advise outside of medical guidelines.

Treating MS by changing your lifestyle is not a

common treatment. That is why a neurologist will generally not advise you on this. This (unfortunately) also makes sense, because a neurologist only knows a lot about the nervous system. However, in a manner of speaking they know as much as you and I do about the effect of nutrition, sports and meditation on the course of MS. In addition, they will be inclined to say that nothing has been proven (although they may have no expertise in this area).

1. That something has not been proven can mean many different things:
2. It has not been proven, because we have research that shows that it is not true.
3. It has not been proven, because we have not researched it.
4. It has not been proven, because we do not yet have enough research to demonstrate this (and therefore I cannot prescribe/ recommend it).
5. It has not been proven because I have not read anything about it.

Now, as a patient you always think that the neurologist means number 1, while they may have 2, 3 or 4 in mind. It is important that you remember the above when you mention that you are following the OMS program. It is very demotivating when a doctor says that what you do does not matter, because it has not been proven.

'So, why do you need a neurologist at all?', you may be asking. First of all, they know an awful lot about nervous system diseases, so you can always present them with your symptoms to see if they are MS-related or not. Secondly, you may want to have an MRI scan after one or two years of implementing lifestyle changes. Using an MRI scanner costs a lot of money and only one person can enter the scanner at a time. An MRI scan is usually used in the treatment of MS to see if the treatment (with medication) is working. For example, if you decide not to take any medication, you are strictly speaking not under any medical treatment (you have refused it, as it were), and your neurologist has no need for an MRI scan of your brain or spinal cord[9].

Here is where it pays to have a good relationship with your neurologist. If your neurologist is sympathetic to you, they are more likely to have you undergo an MRI scan without a medical need. Aside from that, your neurologist has probably also become curious about what your MRI will look like.

## Keep in mind

✓ A neurologist is only human.
✓ Only talk about your MS and don't elaborate too much on OMS.
✓ Not proven does not mean false.
✓ With a good relationship you achieve more, for example an MRI.

---

[9] This was explained to me by the head of neurology at Orbis Medical Center in Sittard-Geleen, the Netherlands.

# Excercise

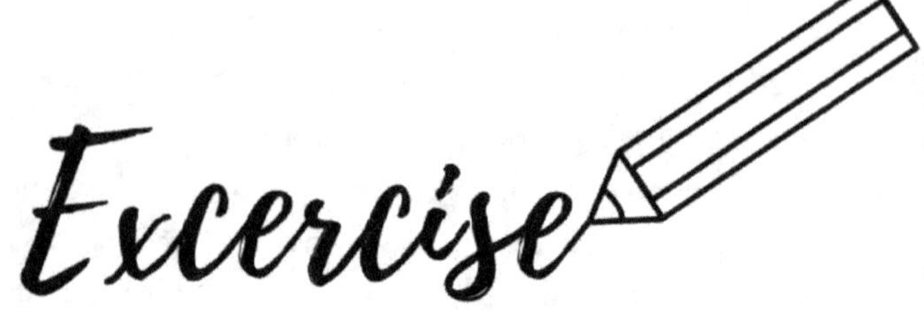

Are you trying to convince your neurologist of the benefits of lifestyle change?

How would you feel if some 'know it all' started to tell you how you should run your business or do your job? No matter if he or she is right.

How would you react?

## Value your MRI scan

I only knew there was a suspicion that I would have MS when the nurse injected contrast fluid into my veins and then let me disappear into the MRI scanner. On the MRI scans that followed, four large MS lesions were found in my brain. A very uncomfortable experience to say the least: You see the inside of your brain and you also see that there are white spots that do not belong there. On the second scan, a year later, all lesions had faded. This gave me great relief; the OMS lifestyle had caught on! Then year three came with the third scan. There were no more of the old lesions to be seen, but a new spot had appeared. Reason for panic? No, because it is 'only' a scan.

An MRI scan is a snapshot of the state of your brain and spinal cord. If you have such a scan at intervals, you can gradually see a trend. That trend means that you usually see more spots in more places. Now it may be that you have a lot of spots and no noticeable symptoms but you can also have very few spots and many symptoms. There is no direct connection between the spots and your symptoms. There is an indirect connection: if you have spots, there is certainly something wrong. What you need to know about this is that with any type of MS, except benign, the attack on your nervous system always continues, even without visible inflammation on the MRI. However, the MRI is used to determine whether your medication is working. The danger that lies in this is that the neurologist will treat according to the MRI scan and not the patient. The drugs decrease the number of visible inflammations (and symptoms), but no drug stops the constant attack on the nervous system. The breakdown therefore always continues. So what is a good indicator?

The best (and most commonly used indicator) is your (changing) spot on the Kurtzke Expanded Disability Status Scale (EDSS)[10]. The EDSS is an indicator for MS that runs from 0 to 10. At 0 there is nothing wrong; you can still do everything and you have no symptoms. With 1 you have a bit of trouble (for example only your vision), with 2 you already have some trouble with moving and a few other symptoms, with 3 this gets worse, and so on up to 10 (death by MS). It's important to remember that if you have been following the OMS program for more than a year and you feel (and move) fit as a fiddle, but an MRI scan shows activity, then there is no reason to panic. It is all about your place on the EDSS. If you went from 3 to 2 after that, because you started living healthier, that is enough reason for celebration. When your MRI supports this image, it is all the better but if your MRI is still showing activity, this is not a disaster. You are not your MRI. It's about where you are on the EDSS[11].

---

[10] See mstrust.org.uk/az/expanded-disability-status-scale-edss

[11] Or as an OMS representative once wrote to me once: it's about how you feel.

## Keep in mind

✓ Don't let your mood depend on the MRI result; it is not an exam.

✓ The main indicator of well-being is the EDSS (0-10).

✓ Make sure your neurologist treats you and not the results of the MRI.

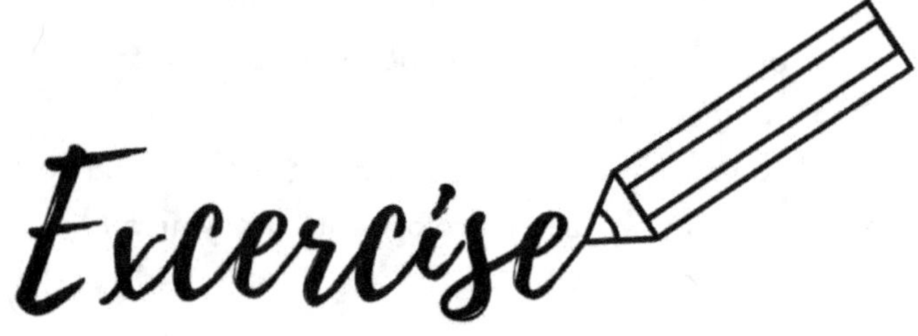

# Excercise

An MRI result can feel like an exam result; how well did I do on OMS until now?

What other ways do you judge yourself and are they of any direct benefit to you managing your MS? Or are you just beating yourself up?

# Ewout's story: the first year after diagnosis

Few things are as drastic and life-altering as the diagnosis of a chronic illness. For me it was in October 2010 just outside the Academic Hospital in Maastricht, the Netherlands. I had just had an MRI scan, where the nurse had said that I was being examined for MS. Riding my bike back home - back then across the nearby border in Belgium - my life just collapsed. I felt powerless, sad and insecure. Why did this have to happen to me? Had I not already experienced enough rottenness in my life? Yet it was already clear to me then: I won't stand for this.

In the time after the MRI, a colleague talked about a diet that might benefit. I went online searching and wounded up through an article about the Swank Diet at the Overcoming Multiple Sclerosis website. I went over everything. If there was an opportunity not to live with the effects of MS, this must be it. The day of preliminary diagnosis, a few weeks after the MRI scan, thus became the starting point of my OMS journey. I cleared my fridge, ate my last hamburger and was completely ready in less than two days. All the while I was still suffering from the after effects of a heavy MS attack. Running was no longer possible and I was tired all the time. In the meantime, I also started to tell the news to my loved ones.

I told my friends and close family that I had been diagnosed with MS, but that a diet had proven to be effective and that it would work out. My friends responded either with support or reluctance. Often the latter were the people who had studied medicine or health sciences. My mother and father were quite scared about it and my sister was completely taken aback. My sister had also invited herself to go through the entire process of definitive diagnosis at Orbis Medical Center in Sittard-Geleen, the Netherlands. VEP, lumbar puncture (which failed every time), blood test; I went through it all with resignation. I developed a shame for my newly 'won' disease. The big surprise when I returned home was that my sister would also stay the night. I found it all uncomfortable and really wanted to be left alone (but now I say thank you, Jen!).

My first appointment with my new neurologist was difficult and would set the tone for the next appointments over the years. With the help of the book Overcoming Multiple Sclerosis, I had thoroughly read up on the matter and I made it known. I told him that given Swank's research results, I would wait a year before taking drugs. He replied that in my place he would be sorry if he could no longer eat chips and as an afterthought if I was interested in participating in a drug trial. Months later, I saw in the national transparency register for medics that in two years (2012-13) he had already earned 13,448 euros with lectures and advice for the manufacturers whose medicines he advocated 'independently' in the newspaper and in the treatment room.

The medicine talk with the nurse was not exactly pleasant either. It seemed more like a bad sales pitch with phrases like, 'most people choose to inject this in the evening, after which they take a handful of aspirins so to sleep through the side effects.' It didn't sound appealing, not least because all medications have been shown to only fight symptoms; they don't stop the progress of MS. When I informed the nurse that I had already chosen not to take medication, she was not exactly charmed by my decision.

After the talk, I went to the MS patients association room in the hospital. All patients appeared to have a firm belief in their treatment and had already accepted their fate. It was the first and last time I would pop by. In the months that followed, I struggled to find new recipes and adjust my eating habits. This was not only a spiritual challenge. Physically, my digestion had to make a transition that was accompanied by a lot of gas. Fortunately, I worked in an old building with faulty sewage, which was often blamed.

I would get two more attacks the first year of my MS. With the first, I called the MS nurse in a slight panic to make an appointment. However, a few hours later I called and canceled. Getting into a conversation would mean talking about medicine. Medicine I didn't want to take during the first year. It would make no sense, she admitted. The second attack was during a salsa class. Every time I had to turn my dance partner around I felt an electric shock in my spine. That evening I felt defeated. How could this be? Shouldn't this 'diet' work? After class I went out with my friends and I danced the attack away with a lot of beer - no salsa by the way, because I wasn't very good at that.

The first year was also characterized by many responses to questions from my peers: 'Why do you eat like this?'; 'Are you vegetarian or something?'; 'Oh really? I couldn't give up bacon!'; 'But you can't live without milk, can you?' And so on. The first cracks in friendships also arose. I still went on weekend trips with my fraternity twice every year, where the social cement consisted of an abundance of fatty foods, sturdy drinking and smoking cigars. Suddenly I did not participate with two of the three by default and without a substantial meal first, you can forget about drinking a lot. In addition, the discussions about these matters had suddenly become a lot less interesting. Also the first gossips started to surface that my new lifestyle was nonsense.

After about a year of OMS, I underwent an MRI scan which was generally very positive. The four large lesions identified in the first MRI were significantly faded. However, there was a new lesion on my brainstem[12]. Better news, however, was that the attack I had had every year in late summer had failed to materialize. Slowly but surely it came to me that OMS really worked and that the theory was becoming practice. The aforementioned salsa attack turned out to be my last attack. In the second year, my residual complaints got less, just like in the third year. After two years of OMS, I underwent another MRI scan. Although the original spots were almost no longer visible, a large spot had appeared. Normally that would indicate an attack, but it hasn't appeared. How you feel is the best

---

[12] For the images see envoeding.eu/uncategorized/mijn-mri-uitslag-2011-in-vergelijking-met-2010

indication of your health, as the moderator of the OMS forum once wrote to me. The scan images did provide a more realistic picture: my MS remains active, but the OMS lifestyle means that the disease cannot do anything. You could say that it is latent or that I am in permanent remittance.

In the time that followed, I felt fitter by the day. I dared to run long stretches again and dream of a future. Soon my eye fell on foreign countries. After saving some money, I moved to Barcelona with my then girlfriend of three years. After a few weeks in the Catalan capital, it already became clear that we no longer had a future together. The period that followed was very difficult for me. I was forced to return to flat-sharing, missed my old environment and friends, worked around the clock and slept too little. You would say the ideal circumstance for an attack, but it never materialized.

After eight months in Barcelona I gave up and started traveling. My idea was after a short stop in Sweden to travel to the Balkans and from there to the Mediterranean Sea, only I never got further than Romania. In Barcelona I had developed a taste for extreme sports. I wanted to crown it with a kayaking course in a wild, Romanian mountain river. The course ended for me when my kayak capsized and my face hit a rock underwater. As a result of the accident, my eyelid was torn and my nose broken. After a rehabilitation period, I returned to the Netherlands for two months, but I had already decided to move to Romania for a while for the incredible nature that the country has to offer. That was five years ago and I still live there today.

Research shows that the longer you don't have an

attack, the less likely it is that you will have one. I had my last attack over nine years ago. Prior to starting with OMS, I had had one at least every six months. I have no idea what the future holds, but statistically, an attack seems unlikely. If I do have one, I am at least grateful for all the time that I have been able to live in good health.

*Frequently asked questions & answers*

Cooking and eating

### Which pans can I use for fat-free cooking?
Basically all types of pans, as long as the pan does not overheat. In pans with a Teflon layer, overheating leads to the release of harmful substances.
*Recommended devices:* blender / food processor, oven, ceramic pan.
*Nice to have:* air fryer, spiralizer, tagine.

### Where can I find recipes?
Besides the Overcoming Multiple Sclerosis Cookbook and ditto website, you can google 'fat free vegan' for delicious recipes. You will also have to make some adjustments, but the recipes form a good base from which to create meals. Also try vegan Italian recipes or with fish.

### Can I heat extra virgin olive oil?
You can use extra virgin olive oil for oven dishes if the oil is used inside the preparation. In the pan you may use a few drops of the extra virgin olive oil. Add a little water

to keep the temperature of the oil down (below 180 C / 405 F).

## What if something contains 0.1 grams of saturated fat per serving, for example 'with pieces of chocolate'?

It is of course better not to, but 0.1 grams of saturated fat is negligible in my view. If you eat 10 servings right away, it's a different story. Do not take this as a rule. It must remain a real exception.

## What do I do if I have accidentally eaten something 'wrong'?

It doesn't make much sense to feel bad about this for a long time. It happens. The best thing to do is learn from it so you don't make the mistake in the future.

## What should I not eat?

For example, the following foods are not part of OMS, so you should avoid them:
- Meat, including processed meat, salami, sausage, canned meat;
- Egg yolk. Egg whites are okay;
- Dairy products. So avoid milk, cream, butter, ice cream and cheeses. Low-fat milk or yogurt is also not acceptable. Soy products, rice or oat milk are good substitutes.
- Biscuits, pastries, cakes, muffins, or donuts, unless fat-free;
- Commercially baked goods;

- Packet sauces and the like from the supermarket;
- Snacks, such as chips, corn chips, birthday snacks;
- Margarine, shortening, lard, chocolate, coconut and palm oil. Cocoa is possible.
- Fried and deep fried foods.
- Most fast food, such as burgers, roasted chicken, and so on;
- Modified fats and oils;
- Coconut.

## Vitamins and medication

### How do you determine your required vitamin intake?

It is a process of trying. I took 5000 IU of vitamin D3 a day for a while, but this was not enough for me to achieve optimal value, so I doubled the dose. To determine your D3 value, have your blood tested with your doctor or in the hospital. In addition, it is also useful to know your vitamin B12 value. The optimal vitamin D3 blood value as recommended by OMS starts at 150 nmol / L or 65 ng/mL.

### Which vitamins are best?

I have never noticed a difference in the quality of vitamin D3 tablets. I personally always buy tablets of 5000 IU online, paying attention to the casing of the capsule (no oil) and the fillers used. I prefer tablets that are sold as vegan / kosher.

### How often do you take vitamins?

Every day I take two tablets of vitamin D3 of 5000IU each. I sometimes skip this when I go sunbathing for a part of the day. I also take a B12 tablet once or twice a week in the weeks that I don't eat fish.

### What can you advise regarding medications?

I never took medication, so I can't advise you on this. Be aware that no drugs on the market have been proven to stop MS or prevent decline.

### Can I take flaxseed or fish oil in hand luggage on a plane?

Normally you can easily take the capsules with you in the plastic bag for the liquids.

### How should you store flaxseed oil and can you cook with it?

You keep the oil in the refrigerator. I try to buy the bottles in stores where they are not exposed to too much light and heat. You cannot heat the oil. Therefore it is not suitable for cooking.

### How much flaxseed oil do you take?

In the beginning I took fish oil capsules but I switched when a study showed that flaxseed oil is slightly better absorbed by your body. I took two tablespoons a day for a long time, but when I noticed I was still fatigued, I started taking three tablespoons. Currently I take two tablespoons a day because I no longer cycle to work. I take three tablespoons on the days that I exercise.

### Are you not protein deficient?
Your body makes the proteins it needs itself. For this it combines, for example, parts of vegetable proteins. Fish is also packed with protein.

### Are you not deficient in calcium, now that you have to avoid dairy?
Calcium is not only found in dairy products, but also in fruit and vegetables. Green vegetables especially, are full of it.

### If I don't take omega-6 oil, will I get enough?
Do not worry. Omega-6 is present in our daily foods such as nuts, seeds, grains and the products that are prepared from them, such as bread and pasta.

## Other

### After how long did OMS catch on with you?
After three months I already noticed some relief from my symptoms. My attacks stopped after nine months. It just takes time.

### Where can I find other OMS followers?
Search on Facebook for OMS or overcoming multiple

sclerosis. OMS also has a forum on their website.

### Did I have an attack?

You should check this with your neurologist. In general, an attack is really tangible. If you have strong doubts, it is probably not an attack. For example, I myself experienced tingling for years after running. Ultimately it turned out that these were caused by trapped nerves.

### Can I deduct costs for OMS from the tax?

Most countries offer the possibility to deduct medical costs including for medical diets. Your tax authority will require your GP to fill in a form. This form will then serve as proof to deduct a lump sum from your income. To support my request to the GP, I took the OMS book and two articles (by Swank in The Lancet[13] and the most recent by Jelinek[14]) with me at the time.

### More questions?

Send me an email! evde@envoeding.eu.

---

[13] See thelancet.com/diarys/lancet/article/PII0140-6736(90)91533-G/fulltext

[14] See ncbi.nlm.nih.gov/pmc/articles/PMC3562546/

## Annex: dinner cards

The cards have been translated by native speakers and language professionals.

### Comments

*Chinese*: the translated text is in Mandarin.
*Korean:* the text has been translated into South Korean, but is also be understandable in North Korea.

*Spanish, Portuguese, Romanian, Czech*: The translation also mentions the preference for pasta, bread and rice varieties, which are whole wheat.

*Turkish*: The Turkish language has no word for 'nuts'. The translator therefore uses a usual description.

*Persian*: The translator reported that cold pressed oil is hard to come by in Iran.

Hello!

I follow a strict medical diet. Are you able to cook me something?

I can't eat products with:

- Processed / refined oils
- Meat
- Dairy (milk, butter, etc)
- Egg yolk
- (Deep) fried foods
- Coconut

I can have, among others:

- ✓ Fish
- ✓ Vegetables, fruit, nuts
- ✓ Pasta, bread, rice
- ✓ Extra virgin olive oil
- ✓ Other cold-pressed oils

Possible modes of preparation:

- ✓ Grilled, in the oven, steamed, boiled

Thank you!

مرحبا

بامكانك هى جدا، وخاص قاس حمية نظام اتبع اذا عليه؟ بناء لي شيء بطهي تقوم ان الامط بوخة الاطعمة اتناول ان استطيع لا يمكنني لا كما، والمعالج المكرر بالزيت

بتناول:

- اللحوم
- حليب زبدة، جبن،)الالبان منتجات (الخ..
- البيض صفار
- كبير بشكل المقلية الاطعمة
- الهند جوز

اخرى اشياء بين من اتناول ان استطيع

✔ باذواعه السمك
✔ والفواكه الخضراوات
✔ والخبز والمعكرونة الارز
✔ والبكر الصافي الزيتون زيت
✔ الباردة الزيوت بعض

لي الممكنة التحضير طريقة

✔ البخار على، الفرن في،الشواية على المغلي

شكرا لك

Здравейте!

Следвам строга медицинска диета. Дали бихте могли да сготвите нещо за мен?

Не мога консумирам следните продукти:

- Преработени/ рафинирани масла
- Месо
- Млечни продукти (мляко, масло и т.н.)
- Жълтък
- (Дълбоко) пържени храни
- Кокос

Сред продуктите, които мога да консумирам са:

✓ Риба
✓ Зеленчуци, плодове, ядки
✓ Спагети, хляб, ориз
✓ Студено пресован зехтин Extra Virgin
✓ Други студено пресовани масла

Възможни начини на обработка:

✓ На скара, Във фурна, Задушени
  Варени

Благодаря!

您好！

我有个严格的医疗饮食。 您可以做饭给我吃吗？

我不可以吃下面的东西：

- 加工/精制的油
- 肉
- 乳制品（牛奶，黄油等）
- 蛋黄
- （深）油炸食品
- 椰子

我可以吃：

- ✓ 鱼
- ✓ 蔬菜，水果，坚果
- ✓ 面食，面包，米饭
- ✓ 特级初榨橄榄油
- ✓ 其他冷榨油

可以吃的方式：

- ✓ 烧烤的, 放在烤箱里的, 蒸的, 煮的

谢谢！

Dobrý den,

dodržuji přísnou lékařskou dietu. Můžete mi prosím připravit nějaké jídlo?

Nemohu jíst následující potraviny:

- Zpracovaný/rafinovaný olej

- Maso

- Mléčné výrobky (mléko, máslo atd.)

- Vaječný žloutek

- Smažená jídla

- Kokos a kokosové deriváty

Mohu mimo jiné jíst:

- ✓ Ryby

- ✓ Zeleninu, ovoce, ořechy

- ✓ Těstoviny (nejlépe bezvaječné), chléb (nejlépe celozrnný), rýži (nejlépe celozrnnou)

- ✓ Extra panenský olivový olej

- ✓ Ostatní oleje lisované za studena

Možné způsoby přípravy:

- ✓ Na grilu, v troubě, v páře, vařené

Děkuji Vám!

Hallo!

Ik volg een strikt medisch dieet. Kunt u iets voor mij bereiden?

Ik mag geen producten met:

- Olie die verwerkt / geraffineerd is

- Vlees

- Zuivel (melk, boter, etc)

- Eigeel

- Gefrituurd of gebakken in olie

- Kokosnoot

Ik mag onder andere wel:

✓ Vis

✓ Groenten, fruit, noten

✓ Pasta, brood, rijst

✓ Extra vierge- olijfolie

✓ Andere koudgeperste olie

Mogelijke bereidingswijzen:

✓ Grillen, in de oven, gestoomd, gekookt

Dank u wel!

Moi!

Noudatan tiukkaa lääketieteellistä ruokavaliota. Pystytkö keittämään minulle jotain?

En voi syödä tuotteita, jotka sisältävät:

- Prosessoitua/puhdistettua öljyä

- Lihaa

- Maitotuotteita (maito, voi jne.)

- Keltuaista

- Paistettuja ruokia

- Kookospähkinää

Voin syödä muun muassa:

- ✓ Kalaa

- ✓ Vihanneksia, hedelmiä, pähkinöitä

- ✓ Pastaa, leipää, riisiä

- ✓ Ekstra neitsyt-oliiviöljyä

- ✓ Muuta kylmäpuristettua öljyä

Mahdollisia valmistustapoja:

- ✓ Grillillä, uunissa, höyryssä, vedessä

Kiitos!

Bonjour!

Je suis un régime médical très strict de nutrition. Êtes-vous capable de me cuisiner quelque chose?

Je ne peux pas manger de produits avec:

- Huiles transformées / raffinées
- Viande
- Produits laitiers (lait, beurre, etc.)
- Jaune d'œuf
- Aliments très frits
- Noix de coco

Je peux manger entre autres:

- ✓ Poisson
- ✓ Légumes, fruits, noix
- ✓ Pâtes, pain, riz
- ✓ Huile d'olive extra vierge
- ✓ Autre huile pressée à froid

Les modes de préparation possibles sont:

- ✓ Sur le grill, dans le four, a la vapeur, bouilli

Merci beaucoup!

Hallo!

ich folge einer strengen medizinischen Diät. Könnten Sie etwas für mich kochen?

Folgende Lebensmittel darf ich nicht essen:

- Behandelte und raffinierte Öle
- Fleisch
- Milchprodukte (Milch, Butter usw.)
- Eigelb
- Frittiertes/Gebratenes
- Kokosnuss

Folgende Lebensmittel darf ich essen:

✓ Fisch
✓ Gemüse, Obst, Nüsse
✓ Nudeln, Brot, Reis
✓ Natives Olivenöl extra
✓ Andere kaltgepresste Öle

Mögliche Zubereitungsarten:

✓ Gegrillt, im Ofen gebacken, dampfgegart, gekocht

Vielen Dank!

Γειά σας !

Ακολουθώ μια αυστηρή διατροφή για ιατρικούς λόγους. Θα μπορούσατε να μου μαγειρέψετε κάτι?

Δε μπορώ να φάω προιόντα που περιέχουν:

- επεξεργασμένο λάδι
- κρέας
- γαλακτοκομικά (γάλα, βούτυρο κτλ)
- κρόκος αυγού
- τηγανητά φαγητά
- καρύδα

Μπορώ να καταναλώσω μεταξύ άλλων:

- ✓ ψάρι
- ✓ λαχανικά, φρούτα, ξηρούς καρπούς
- ✓ μακαρόνια, ψωμίι, ρύζι
- ✓ έξτρα παρθένο ελαιόλαδο
- ✓ άλλο ψυχρό έλαιο

Πιθανοί τρόποι παρασκευής:

- ✓ στο γκριλ, στο φούρνο, στον ατμό, βραστά

Ευχαριστώ πολύ!

नमस्कार!

मैं चिकित्सा कारणों से सीमित आहार का पालन करता हूं।

क्या आप मेरे लिए कुछ पका सकते हैं?

मैं निम्नलिखित उत्पादों के साथ कुछ भी नहीं खा सकता हूं:

- तेल जो संसाधित / परिष्कृत होते हैं
- मांस
- डेयरी (दूध, मक्खन, आदि)
- अंडे की जर्दी
- तले हुए खाद्य पदार्थ
- नारियल

मैं निम्नलिखित उत्पादों को खा सकता हूं:

✓ मछली
✓ सब्जियां, फल, नट
✓ पास्ता, रोटी, चावल
✓ अतिरिक्त शुद्ध जैतून का तेल
✓ अन्य प्राकृतिक तेल

तैयारी के संभावित तरीके:

✓ तंदूर पर, ओवन में, भाप से तैयार, उबला हुआ

धन्यवाद!

Helló!

Egy igen szigorú, orvosi diétát követek. Tudna/Tudnál nekem valamit készíteni?

- Nem ehetek termékeket, amik a következőket tartalmazzák:

- Finomított étolaj

- Hústejtermék (tej, vaj, stb.)

- Tojássárgája

- Olajban kisütött ételek

- Kókusz

A következőket ehetem:

✓ Halak

✓ Zöldségek, gyümölcsök, diófélék

✓ Tésztafélék, kenyérfélék, rizs

✓ Extra szűz olívaolaj

✓ Egyéb hidegen préselt olajok

Az előkészítés lehetséges módjai:

✓ grillezve, sütőben sütve, párolva, főzve

Köszönöm!

Ciao!

Sto seguendo una particolare dieta medica. Sapresti cucinare alcune cose per me?

Io non posso mangiare prodotti con:

- — Olio raffinato

- — Carne

- — Latticini (latte, burro ecc.)

- — Tuorlo d'uovo

- — Fritture

- — Cocco

Posso invece mangiare:

- ✓ Pesce

- ✓ Verdure, frutta e noci

- ✓ Pasta, pane e riso

- ✓ Olio extra vergine di oliva,

- ✓ Altri olii a spremutura a freddo.
  Possibili cotture:

- ✓ Arrosto, al forno, al vapore, bollitura

Grazie!

こんにちは。

私の食生活に関して、注意する点が多くあります。以下を参照の上、調理をお願いできますか？

食べられない物：

- 精製　加工植物油（マーガリン、ショートニング、サラダ油、一般的な植物油など）
- 肉
- 乳製品（牛乳、バターなど）
- 卵の黄身
- 揚げ物
- ココナッツ

食べられる物：

- ✓ 魚
- ✓ 野菜、果物、ナッツ
- ✓ パスタ、パン、米
- ✓ エクストラバージンオリーブオイル
- ✓ その他の冷たい圧搾製法植物油

問題の無い調理方法：

- ✓ グリルで焼く，オーブンで焼く，蒸す，ゆでる、煮る

お手数をお掛けしますが、どうぞよろしくお願いします。

안녕하세요!

저는 엄격한 의료 식단을 따르고 있습니다.

저를 위해 요리해주실 수 있으십니까?

제가 먹을 수 없는 식재료는 다음과 같습니다:

- 가공유 및 정제유

- 육류

- 유제품 (우유, 버터 등)

- 계란 노른자

- (기름에 잠기게 하여) 튀긴 음식

- 코코넛

제가 먹을 수 있는 식재료는 다음과 같습니다:

- ✓ 생선

- ✓ 채소, 과일, 견과류

- ✓ 파스타, 빵, 쌀

- ✓ 엑스트라 버진 올리브유

- ✓ 기타 냉압착유

가능한 조리 방식은 다음과 같습니다:

- ✓ 석쇠, 오븐, 찜, 가열

감사합니다!

Hello!

Saya mengikuti diet perubatan yang ketat, adakah anda boleh memasak saya sesuatu?

Saya tidak boleh makan makanan yand mengandungi:

- — Minyak diproces
- — Daging
- — Produk tenusu (susu, mentega dan lain lain)
- — Kuning telur
- — Makanan goreng dalam
- — Kelapa

Saya boleh makan makanan berikut:

- ✓ Ikan
- ✓ Sayur-sayuran, buah-buahan, kacang
- ✓ Pasta, roti dan beras
- ✓ Minyak zaitun Extra Virgin
- ✓ Minyak yang melalui perahan sejuk

Cara penyediaan yang mungkin:

- ✓ Panggang, di dalam ketuhar, mengewap, direbus

Terima Kasih

Heisan!

Jeg følger en streng medisinsk diett. Kan du lage noe mat til meg?

Jeg kan spise matvarer som:

- Behandlet oljer/raffinerte oljer
- Kjøtt
- Meieriprodukter (melk, smør, etc)
- Eggeplomme
- Fritert mat
- Kokosnøtt

Blant annet, kan jeg spise:

✓ Fisk

✓ Grønnsaker, frukt, nøtter

✓ Makaroni, brød, ris

✓ Extra virgin olivenolje

✓ Andre typer kaldpresset olje

Mulige kokemetoder:

✓ Grillet, i ovnen, dampkokt, kokt

Takk!

روز خیر .یـ

غذای یـ رژیـ م یـ ک بـ ندہ پـ ز شک، د سـ تور طـ بق این در مـ یـ توذ یـد .کـ نم دذ بال بـ ایـ د درو سخت کـ ذ یـد؟ کـ مـ کم زمـ یـنه

من مـ یـ توانـ مـ یـ ذمـ ی غذاهلیـ بـ ا مواد ر زیـ را خورم بـ:

— روغن هلی غـ نیـ شدہ

— گـ و شت

— لـ بـ ذ یـات (غـ یرہ و شـ یر،کـ رہ،)

— مرغ تـ خم زردہ

— غذاهای سرخ شدہ (زیـ اد روغن در)

— یـل ذ ارگـ

مـ یـ توانـ مـ را زیـ ر غذاهای: بـ خورم، کـ ه تـ بـ ال محدود بـ:
بـ یـست لـ یـست این بـ ه.

✓ ماهی

✓ آجـ یل و هـ سـ بزیـ جات،مـ یوه

✓ بـ زنذ جـ ذ ان، ماکـ ارانـ یـ،

✓ فـ راب کـ ر طـ بـ یـعی زیـ تون روغن

✓ طـ بـ یـعی هلی روغن دیـ گرو

انـ واع خـ تی پـ کـ ه لـ قابـ ق بول قـ شدند بـ ا مـ یـ:

✓ بـ خارپـ ز ,گـ ذاشتن فـ ر در ,کـ ردن گـ ریـ ل

جو شاذدن

ا مـ مـ نون

Olá!

Eu sigo uma dieta médica estrita. Você pode preparar algo para mim?

Eu não posso comer:

— Óleo que é processado / refinado

— Carne

— Laticínios (leite, manteiga, etc)

— Gema de ovo

— Alimentos fritos

— Coco e derivados do coco

Eu posso, entre outras coisas comer:

✓ Peixe

✓ Legumes, frutas, nozes

✓ Massas (de preferencia sem ovo), pão (de preferencia integral), arroz (de preferencia integral)

✓ Azeite virgem extra

✓ Outros óleos prensados a frio

Possíveis métodos de preparação:

✓ Grelhar, no forno, cozido no vapor, cozido

Obrigado!

Bună ziua!

Urmez o dietă medicală strictă. Îmi puteți pregăti ceva de mâncare?

Nu pot mânca:

- Ulei prelucrat / rafinat
- Carne
- Produse lactate (lapte, unt etc.)
- Gălbenuș de ou
- Mâncare prăjită
- Cocos și derivați de nucă de cocos

Pot, printre altele, să mănânc:

- ✓ Pește
- ✓ Legume, fructe, nuci
- ✓ Paste (de preferat fără ou), pâine (de preferință integrală), orez (de preferință integral)
- ✓ Ulei de măsline extravirgin
- ✓ Alte uleiuri presate la rece

Metode de preparare posibile:

- ✓ La grătar, la cuptor, la abur, fierbere

Mulțumesc!

Здравствуйте!

У меня очень строгая диета по медицинским причинам. Смогли бы Вы приготовить мне что-нибудь?

Я не могу употреблять такие продукты как:

- Рафинированное масло
- Мясо
- Молочные и кисломолочные продукты
- Яичный желток
- Жареную пищу
- Кокос

Продукты которые я могу употреблять:

✓ Рыба
✓ Овощи, фрукты, орехи
✓ Макароны, хлеб, рис
✓ Оливковое масло первого отжима
✓ Другие масла холодного отжима

Возможные способы приготовления:

✓ На гриле, В духовке, На пару, вареный

Большое спасибо!

¡Hola!

Sigo una dieta médica estricta. ¿Puede prepararme algo?

No puedo comer:

- Aceite procesado / refinado
- Carne
- Productos lácteos (leche, mantequilla, etc.)
- Yema de huevo
- Alimentos fritos
- Coco y derivados del coco

Puedo, entre otras cosas, comer:

- ✓ Pescado
- ✓ Verduras, frutas, nueces
- ✓ Pasta (preferiblemente sin huevo), pan (preferiblemente integral), arroz (preferiblemente integral)
- ✓ Aceite de oliva virgen extra
- ✓ Otros aceites prensados en frío

Posibles métodos de preparación:

- ✓ Asar a la parrilla, en el horno, al vapor, cocido

¡Gracias!

Merhaba!

Benim ozel tibbi bir beslenmem var. Benim icin uygun yemek pişirebilir misiniz?

İçinde aşağıdaki ürünler bulunan yemekleri yiyemiyorum:

- İşlenmiş veya rafine edilmiş yağ
- Et ürünleri
- Süt ürünleri (süt, tereyağı, vb.)
- Yumurta Sarısı
- Kızartma yemekler
- Hindistan cevizi

Yiyebilecegim gidalar:

- ✓ Balık
- ✓ Sebze, meyve, fındık, fıstık
- ✓ Makarna, ekmek, pirinç
- ✓ Gercek islenmemis soğuk pres sızma zeytinyağı
- ✓ Diger soğuk pres islenmemiş yağlar

Pişirme şekli:

- ✓ Yağsız ızgara, fırında, buğulama, haşlama

Teşekkürler!

Hej!

Jag följer en strikt medicinsk diet. Klarar du att laga något åt mig?

Jag kan inte äta produkter med:

- Oljor som bearbetas / raffineras

- kött

- Mejeri (mjölk, smör, etc)

- Äggula

- (Djupt) stekt mat

- Kokosnöt

Jag kan ha bland annat:

- ✓ Fisk

- ✓ Grönsaker, frukt, nötter

- ✓ Pasta, bröd, ris

- ✓ Extra virgin-olivolja

- ✓ Andra kallpressade oljor

Möjliga sätt att "förbereda" maten:

- ✓ På grillen, i ugnen, ångad, kokt

Tack!

Liked the book? Please leave a review.


78

*About the author*

Dutch born Ewout van den Engel (1983) graduated from Maastricht University, the Netherlands, where he studied science from a cultural perspective. At the age of 27, he was diagnosed with relapsing-remitting multiple sclerosis, after which he started the Overcoming Multiple Sclerosis lifestyle. Since then, Ewout has been blogging about his new lifestyle, including as a guest blogger on overcomingmultiplesclerosis.org (2019 / 2020) and manonamsion.wordpress.com (2011) under the pen name MSmingle.

Ewout also holds a certificate in Plant Based Nutrition from T. Collin Campbell Center for Nutrition Studies. After more than six years of following OMS, he took the plunge and moved abroad. Ewout lived briefly in Spain and has been living in the Romanian capital Bucharest since his move there in 2016, where he lives together with his girlfriend. In addition to his profession as a writer on cultural differences, Ewout also has time for hiking in the mountains and running. Ewout no longer has any (residual) symptoms.